Effective Natural Constipation Cures For Women

"If you are pregnant or not here are the best natural constipation remedies"

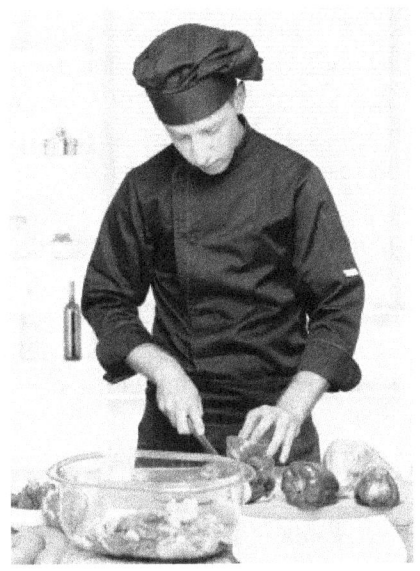

Rudy Silva, Natural Nutritionist

Effective Natural Constipation Cures For Women © 2013 by Rudy S Silva

ISBN-13: 978-1482548280
ISBN-10: 1482548283

Printed in the United States of America

Table of Contents

Introduction

Seventy percent or more of the population struggles with constipation. Some believe the number is even higher like 80-90%. And, there are more women than men who become constipated.

So why is this? Well, women have more stress in their lives. They have to deal with work and home life, their bodies depend more on hormones, and they have babies.

And in many cases, women tend not to use public bathrooms for bowel movements and will hold back on their bowel urges. This practice tends to train the colon not to have a bowel movement after the first urge comes. When you get the urge, you should go to the bathroom soon.

When women are pregnant, they have more difficulty in having a bowel movement, because they have increased pressure on the colon from the growth of their baby. After giving birth, the colon can still be affected by the long birth process and needs to regain its normal function. But, in some cases, women will still have constipation and need to learn how to get back to normal.

There are many other reasons why women have more constipation than men and whatever that reason is this e-book will give you a process where you can eliminate constipation. The ideas in the e-book will help to normalize your whole-body system and gain some health back.

This e-book is not just about getting rid of your constipation. It is about using nutrition to eliminate constipation and at the same time help you gain more health.

As a nutritionist, I consider constipation a serious problem, even though you might get constipated once in a while. The reason is most people don't know what constipation is and how to identify when their colon is not working properly. I believe that many people are constipated and don't know it.

I recommend that when you become constipated, you try to identify why this has occurred. If you can do this, then you can take the right action to eliminate it. Is It because you have started taking medical drugs, changed your diet, not eating enough fiber, eating too much processed food, or going through some emotional issue?

In, Natural Alternatives to Over-the-Counter and Prescription Drugs, 1994, Michael T. Murray, N.D. says,

"Since the frequency of defecation and the consistency and volume of stools vary so greatly from individual to individual, it is difficult to determine what is normal.

Nonetheless, most nutritionally oriented physicians consider two to three bowel movements each day as ideal. This is the number that is typically found in healthy people eating a high-fiber diet and getting adequate exercise."

1: The Truth about Drugstore Laxatives

One client of mine told me she was on drugstore laxatives for over a year and could not have a bowel movement without using them. Laxatives are addictive and cause your colon to become inactive. They also interfere with the amount of minerals you absorb and can cause you to become deficient in specific minerals.

Don't let this happen to you. You are at the right spot right now to learn what you need to do about your constipation.

If you have been using laxative and can't have a bowel movement without them, you will have to retrain your colon to have bowel movements. This book does not cover this topic. But, you can use the information here to start doing the things that can get your body back to normal and at the same time you need to retrain your colon to activate peristaltic action on its own.

Laxatives work by starting and stimulating peristaltic action. Peristaltic action is a wave-like movement that occurs throughout your gastrointestinal tract – esophagus, stomach, small intestine, and colon – that helps move food into your stomach, through your intestines, through your colon, and out your rectum.

There are specific foods and nutrients that can stimulate peristaltic action more than other foods, and these will be discussed in this book.

Drug Store Products

There are drugstore products, natural occurring foods, herbal, substances, and homeopathic liquids that have laxative effects. I do not recommend using drugstore laxatives or any other form of drugs to clear constipation. Drugs store laxatives cause your colon function abnormally, which will create side effects. Constipation can and is typically cured using natural remedies and techniques.

These are some of the drug store products that you want to avoid:

Alin plus phenolphthalein – Dioctyl sodium sulfosucciante – a detergent type substance that lowers the surface tension of your colon walls and fecal matter.

Magnesium hydroxide – brings in more water into your colon.

Osmolak plus lactulose (lactulose is a synthetic sugar that pulls water out of the body and into your colon to soften stools.)

Sokol plus mineral oil

Dioctyl sodium Sulfosucciante belongs to a family of chemicals that reduces the surface tension of the fecal matter in your colon, allowing water and fat to penetrate and make the fecal matter softer. These chemicals are known as,

Dioctyl sodium succiante (also known as docusate sodium)

Dioctyl potassium succinate (also known as docusate potassium)

Dioctyl calcium succinate (also know as docusate calcium) If you are tempted to use drugstore laxatives remember that, **Laxatives bought in drugstores are of questionable safety, when used long term.**

Because of this action these laxatives have on the small intestine and colon, doctors and other health practitioners recommend their limited use. They, have chemical side effects that,

1. produce an active force that can damage nerves that control the muscles in your colon walls

2. desensitize your colon so your natural peristaltic action is reduced

3. become habit-forming when used for 6 months to a year

4. rush your food through your intestines so it does not digest

5. Affect the absorption of nutrients or minerals

6. kill friendly bacteria

7. contain preservatives, coloring, and other additives that are unhealthy

8. remove excessive fluids and electrolytes from your body.

If you are pregnant, do not use mineral oil or other oils to get relief from constipation. During pregnancy, you need good absorption of minerals to provide nutrients for your newborn. Excessive use of mineral oil during pregnancy can cause bleeding and suck out minerals that need to go into your blood stream.

Doctor and Constipation

If you visit a doctor, your colon is the last area they discuss with you. And perhaps, this is an area they may never discuss with you at all.

*In his article, The Bowel is an Ecosystem, in Healthy &
Natural Journal, April 1997, Majid Ali, M.D. recounts,*

"When I returned to the clinical practice of environmental and
nutritional medicine after years of pathology work, I began
carefully testing the assertions of nutritionists, naturopaths
and clinical ecologist who claimed that various types of colitis
[a deterioration of your colon wall] could be reversed with
optimal nutritional and ecologic approaches.

To my great surprise, I found that such professionals, who are
usually spurned by drug doctors, were right after all. My
patients responded well to the unscientific therapies
vehemently rejected by my colleagues in drug medicine."

By concentrating on eliminating constipation and preserving
colon health, you have taken a major step in preventing many-
body conditions and illnesses that arise from constipation and
poor colon healing. Poor colon health can shorten your life or
make your senior years a miserable time.

It takes some work to get rid of constipation. But, you are
going to be eating, thinking, and living, so why not do it right
and gradually let go of the unhealthy habits. It is your choice.
Now, take the right path. I am here to help you.

2: What Is Constipation?

As stated earlier, if you do not have at least 1 to 2 bowel movements per day, then you are constipated. Some people don't have a movement in 2 to 3 days and for sure they constipated.

Whatever you eat should be digested and processed through your body and colon within 24 hours. If it is taking longer, like two days, then you are at a higher risk for hemorrhoids, varicose veins, diverticulosis and many other diseases.

Food Digestion

One of the critical items that affect how often you have a bowel movement is your digestion. You must have good digestion. If you have acid reflux, stomach gas, indigestion, hiatus hernia, ulcers and other stomach issues, this will affect the normalcy of your bowel movements.

Chewing

So this is a good place to start. First make sure you are chewing your food completely. If you swallow chunks of food that have not been chewed properly, your stomach will not break down this food and it will pass into your colon.

In your colon, this food will putrefy, and it becomes food for bad bacteria, and they multiply. If the bad bacteria overcomes the good bacteria, your colon will start to malfunction and you will be more susceptible to constipation.

Remember your stomach does not have teeth, so chew your food well.

Drinking Water

Limit the amount of liquid that you drink with your meals. By drinking too much water, you dilute your stomach acid and reduce the action of your stomach digestion. This leaves undigested food, which becomes food for bad bacteria.

Drinking less liquid includes sodas, juices, and other liquids. Try not to drink liquids at meal time, but if you have to clear your throat, drink room-temperature water to clear my throat.

Drinking any cold liquid with your mean slows down your digestion process. The longer your food stays in your stomach than is necessary the more digestive problems you will have.

Micro Flora or Probiotic in Your Colon

Bacteria in your colon are referred to by many different names – micro flora, probiotics, good or bad bacteria, beneficial bacteria, acidophilus, disbiosis, proflora, friendly flora, and unfriendly bacteria.

I use the words good and bad bacteria to refer to all the bacteria that exist in the small intestine and your colon.

Your colon has both good and bad bacteria. The good bacteria maintain the health of your colon, by keeping the bad bacteria at bay and from multiplying.
Most people have bad bacteria as the dominant condition in their colon. You can see this by the illnesses that exist throughout the world. Most people, later in their lives, suffer from diseases that resulted from colon neglect and abuse.

Bad bacteria multiples when you,

- Consume poisons such as pollution, pesticides, food additives

- Drink alcohol
- Eat processed foods
- Have excess anxiety
- Lack fiber in your diet
- Use birth control pills
- Use drugstore laxative
- Use drugs and medication

Your colon serves as a home for the good bacteria, which ferment specific carbohydrates, which in turn keep your colon environment slightly acidic. The acid environment favors the good bacteria and keeps the bad bacteria and pathogens from multiplying.

When good beneficial bacteria are dominant in your colon, it prevents the spread of disease from various organisms – parasites, bacteria, viruses, fungi. Some of the organisms are,

Shigella
Salmonella
Viruses
Encephalitis
Protozoan
Amebas
Staph
Herpes
flu and cold viruses
comphylobacter

CMV, which creates killer diseases such as dysentery, blood poisoning, meningitis, pneumonia, influenza and encephalitis.

Good bacteria need to be fed to keep them dominant in your colon. If there are any good bacteria left in your colon, then by feeding them, you can get them to multiply. The good bacteria can help to keep your colon pH acidic.

You can feed the good bacteria by eating these vegetables.

1. Onions – eat at least one medium-sized onion each day. The onion can be eaten cooked or raw.

2. Cabbage – eat cabbage or drink cabbage juice. Drink at least 3/4 cup of cabbage juice 3 times a day and eat at least one pound of fresh organic cabbage each day. This amount is necessary to provide the good bacteria with plenty of food to get it to multiply. Cabbage has an added advantage of suppressing the bad bacteria. Eating any amount of cabbage is helpful

3. Sun Choke or Jerusalem artichokes – eat 4 oz of sun chokes each day. Sun chokes contain a carbohydrate call inulin, which is not digested or absorbed in the small intestine. This allows it to reach your colon where it feeds the good bacteria.

3: Foods That Cause Constipation

Causes of constipation

One of the first things you need to do is to stop doing those things that cause constipation. Look over the different things listed here and start changing the way you eat and the lifestyle you have.

Don't try to stop all of the things listed here all at once or even in a month, that would be impossible to do and if you did you would only hurt yourself with side effects. Just slowly start changing your eating habits. Maybe do a couple things a week. You be the judge of what you can do.

Now add to these changes the things that promote having regular bowel movements. These things are listed in the next chapters. And again make these changes little by little.

Your colon is designed to move undigested matter and various bodily wastes through its tract and out the rectum. It does this naturally only when this matter and waste have bulk, fiber, and water. It is this bulk or fiber that pushes against your colon walls and triggers peristaltic action. You can only get this bulk when you eat plenty of fruits, vegetables, and grains that have a combination of soluble and nonsoluble fiber.

Meat, fish, processed food, and dairy products have little or no fiber. In your colon, these foods do not move easily and remain too long in your colon.

Constipation come from unnatural living

Constipation is a complex symptom that is caused by many conditions that have accumulated in your body and caused your colon to malfunction.

Constipation can be caused by a physical weakness due to surgery, inactivity, or deformities, which were inherited or acquired through injury or surgery. Constipation caused by these conditions can be improved by using natural nutrients and alternative methods.

However, it is more difficult to help constipation resulting from physical weakness, since the physical conditions have to be improved.

The continual use of medications or drugs of any sort can cause constipation. This is one reason why many people who are on drugs and have constipation have a difficult time getting rid of it.

Psychological constipation

Constipation is also related to psychological and emotion issues. Anxiety will cause the nerves, wall tissue and muscles in your colon to tense up or contract. If you have a personality that holds feelings or thoughts inside you and don't discuss them with the people you should, you will mostly likely have continual constipation. In fact, you will also be a candidate for creating a variety of destructive internal conditions.

If you have stresses and anxieties in your life, constipation can be a result. Anxiety can also overwork your adrenal gland making it output cortisol. Overtime, because cortisol is toxic to the brain, cortisol will damage and kill brain cells, which can lead to premature old age and Alzheimer's. You will also feel tired and run down when you over stress your Adrenal.

Sometimes constipation can suddenly appear when changes in normal living habits and stressful conditions have occurred –

flying out of your time zone, having personal confrontations at work or within the family.

Infrequent bouts with constipation are really nothing to worry about and can be corrected by many of the suggestions listed in this book

The main cause of constipation is the continual eating of processed foods, which has little food value or fiber and is packed with poison additives. This results in colon wall weakness, where fecal matter cannot even be push out of the rectum.

Eating food with little or no fiber creates fecal matter that is mushy or hard and compacted. Mushy or compact fecal matter is hard to move along your colon and your colon walls tire after many peristaltic movements. After a time, your colon walls stop trying and you end up with constipation.

Constipation is a body condition you have created by improper living choices, which you can change. It is sometimes an easy symptom to eliminate and at other time difficult to deal with. It occurs from a complex of many things. Like so many other body conditions or illnesses, it is a result of:

- Absorbing too many toxins into the body
- Anxiety and depression
- Being bedridden
- Having colitis, or spastic colon.
- Having diabetes
- Having diseases of the anus or rectum - tumors, diverticulosis
- Drinking coffee
- Drinking milk
- Drinking sodas
- Drinking juices with sugar
- Drinking tea

- Eating excess protein
- Eating food that doesn't have fiber
- Eating processed foods
- Eating sugars
- Eating to much food at one sitting
- Excessive exposure to organophosphate insecticides
- Excessive use iron supplements
- Excessive use of enemas
- Excessive use of seasonings
- Excessive Calcium in the body
- Fatigue
- Food sensitivities
- High fever – colon accumulates heat and hardens stools
- Hypothyroidism - Low levels of thyroid hormone
- Kidney failure
- Lacking good bacteria
- Mineral Deficiency
- Nerve disorders of your bowel
- Not chewing food completely
- Not drinking enough water
- Not enough exercise
- Older people
- Overeating
- Overuse of laxatives
- Overdose of Vitamin D
- Parasites
- Poor digestion
- Postponing a bowel movement
- Pregnancy
- Premenstrual tension

So, you can see that constipation can be caused by a variety of different unhealthy lifestyle practices.

Here is another practice that causes constipation.

Make sure that you don't eat or drink at least 2 1/2 hour before bed time. Your stomach will not have to time to finish digesting this food by bed time. And remember that undigested food causes constipation.

If you have to eat sometime have some fresh squeeze juice or eat some fruit. It takes around 1 1/2 to digest fruits or fruit juices.

4: Preventing Constipation

Preventing constipation will require a change in the way you eat, exercise, and think – a life style change - and this can sometimes be difficult, but it's something good. It requires a new mind-set and plenty of willpower. Don't wait until you have an illness to change your mind-set. If you are ill, then this change is necessary now.

If the lifestyle you lead or if your overuse of drugstore laxatives is producing constipation, then a change is necessary to prevent further constipation. With a lifestyle change, you can expect to have normal bowel movements in 2 to 6 weeks. I'm not going to tell you that you can do it in 3 days or one week.

You will need a life style where you get plenty of fiber, moisture, lubrication, minerals, vitamins, vegetables, fruits, juices, water and exercise to prevent constipation.

Older people have to be more diligent in following good eating habits than those younger. Older people's digestive abilities have slowed down and their peristaltic sensors are less sensitive. For these reasons, MSM is a supplement that they should take regularly - 3000 to 4000 mg per day.

Changes to Make to Prevent Constipation

The following eating habits and lifestyles will help to prevent constipation. Don't try to make all of these changes at once. It is too difficult. Make these changes gradually. Not only will you prevent constipation, but also you will create excellent health.

Drink plenty of water, and it does not have to be eight glasses a day. You have to sense when you are thirsty and drink water then. Your body needs water that comes from fruits, vegetables, fruit or vegetable juices, herbal teas, and just plain distilled water.

- Eat less processed carbohydrates
- Eat more nutritious food
- Eat plenty of fiber
- Eat the good oils
- Reduce emotional upsets – at home, office, and business
- Exercise regularly
- Feed the good bacteria
- Get plenty of rest and sleep
- Keep you colon acidic
- Take a good mineral supplement
- Use digestive enzymes

Drinking Plenty Of Water

The body needs plenty of distilled water every day to eliminate toxins from inside and outside its cells and from the blood. When you don't drink enough water, your body becomes dehydrated and will pull excess water out of your fecal matter in your colon. This causes your fecal matter to become dry and more difficult to move through your colon.

Drinking extra water is not to prevent constipation; it is for preventing you from becoming dehydrated. When you become dehydrated you are subject to many illnesses including constipation.

If you drink more water, it will not move into your colon. The water you drink is absorbed through the small intestine and only a small amount will move into your colon as a lubricant and into the fecal matter.

If your body has plenty of water, it will draw less water from your colon and your fecal matter will not become dry and hard.

Best Water To Drink

What is the best water to drink? Facet water is out. There are three other forms of water to drink – regular bottled water, reverse osmosis (RO) water, and distilled water.

Distilled water is the best water to drink. It is the purest type of water and has all contaminates removed. Despite critics that point out this water can leach out minerals from your body, this water is the best and does not leach out minerals from your body.

But in any case, it is best to vary the water you drink.

It is best to store distilled water in a glass container, if possible. Most plastic containers are made from polycarbonate plastic which contain Bisphenol-A. Bisphenol A has many health issues as shown in clinical studies.

Drink little water with your meal, since excess water will dilute your digestive acid in your stomach. This will reduce your ability to digest protein. Drink water only when food accumulates in your throat.

When you do drink water with your meal, drink room temperature water and notice or cold water. Cold water contracts your stomach and surrounding blood vessels. This will slow down your digestive process.

Drink a minimum of 2 quarts of water each day. Because I don't always like the taste of pure water, I sometimes add a fresh squeezed lemon in one quart of water. In this way, I am able to drink more water, at least two quarts each day. Or, I make a ginger tea to drink in the morning and afternoon and flavor it with a little honey.

To prevent lemon acid water from etching my teeth, I have another jar of water without lemon that I use to rinse and drink from after drinking lemon water.

You can add Alkalife drops to your distilled water. This product turns your water into an electrolyte – mineral water, which has minerals in ionic form. Electrolytes are the type of liquid that surrounds your cells and is capable of neutralizing acids that are harmful to your health.

What is Considered Water?

Liquids or juices that do not have added salt or sugar can be considered water. Water for your body also comes from:

- Fruit juices and fruits
- Herbal teas
- Vegetables, vegetable juices and broths
- Distilled water

Water does not come from:

- Sodas
- Sweeten fruit juices
- Coffee with sugar
- Tea with sugar
- Facet water

Urine Color

Watch the color of your urine. The color should be a light yellow to colorless. If it is a dark yellow, you are not drinking enough water.

The dark color results from the toxins your kidney is removing from your blood. If you are not drinking enough water, toxins become concentrated and color your urine. Over time, this condition will affect the health of your kidney. Notice that when you are sick your urine is a darker yellow, which means you need more nutrition when you are sick.

Also, if you are taking B vitamins your urine will be deep yellow. B vitamins are water soluble and your body excretes the excess.

Eat Less Processed Carbohydrates

The foods you must avoid to prevent constipation and at the same time improve your health are foods that are difficult to move through your colon and that create mucus in your body. These are processed foods, fried foods, and dairy products.

All dry foods such as bread, biscuits, bagels, crackers, bran, powdered foods, are difficult to move through your colon and can lead to constipation.

Processed foods cause constipation, since these foods lack fiber, nutrients, and enzymes. Consider all food products that come in bags, plastic, cans, and other containers processed foods. These foods contain excessive sugars, salt, coloring, dyes, hydrogenated oils, flavor enhancer's, and preservatives, and many other unknown chemicals. These foods have been over baked, pasteurized, homogenized, cured, or killed in a hundred other ways.

These foods lack vitamins, minerals, nutrients, fiber, and life, which have been destroyed by heat, pressure, vacuum, and chemicals. Adding vitamins and minerals back into this food does not make it better, since manufacturers cannot duplicate nature.

The vitamins and minerals, added back into the food, are out of balance and do not have the right quantity. When you eat processed food they require minerals to be digested so they pull those minerals from your body that you need for other health purposes.

Here are some of the foods to avoid:

Alcohol, wine, and caffeine – they dehydrate the body by using up body fluids.

- Processed foods
- Coffee
- Dairy products – eggs, milk, cheese butter
- Fried foods
- Excess meat
- Raisin Bran
- Refined sugar
- Regular tea – Tea is rich in tannins, which are helpful for diarrhea but act to hold back bowel movements.
- Salt
- Sodas
- Starch
- Sweets
- Cooked eggs, pasteurized milk, overcooked meat
- Mashed potatoes with gravy
- Overcooked carbohydrates
- Lipton or black Tea

Coffee and tea have a tightening affect – astringent – on your colon and this produces constipation. Drinking coffee on some occasions will have the opposite effect and can promote a bowel movement.

Coffee or tea is not a recommended drink when you have constipation or when you are trying to prevent constipation. This is not true of most herbal teas, which do not contain caffeine.

The caffeine can be found in,

Ground percolated coffee, 8 oz -------- 200 mg
Brewed tea, 8 oz ----------------------- 75 mg
Soft drinks ------------------------------- 40 mg
Chocolate -------------------------------- 10 – 40 mg
Painkillers -------------------------------- 60 mg

Fried Foods

Eating meat, bacon, sausage, and other fatty foods is constipating. These foods and others like butter, cheese, eggs provide an excess of saturated fat and cholesterol that can easily stick to your colon walls. Cholesterol clings to your colon walls just as it does in your arteries.

Meat

All kinds of meat are free fiber, and this makes them constipating. Meat moves slower through your colon than other foods. Since people eat a lot of meat at one sitting, undigested proteins usually make their way into your colon, which is fermented by bad bacteria. This decay creates a condition favorable for bad bacteria and is the start of many diseases that occur in your colon.

It is always best to eat plenty of uncooked vegetables when eating meat, carbohydrates or other food that contains no fiber. This provides fiber to help the food you eat to move quicker through your colon.

Milk and Other Dairy Products

Dairy products are associated with constipation. This includes milk, cream soups, cheese, yogurt, and some desserts and baked goods. The best dairy product to eat is cottage cheese. It is the least harmful to the body of all dairy products.

Eggs

Eggs, cheese, and butter are constipating and form toxic wastes, which poison the body. These foods can be eaten, but minimize their use.

Sodas

Soft drinks are high in phosphates. This chemical is used to dissolve sugar and to make soda taste better. When you drink soda, the phosphates combine with calcium. If you do not have enough calcium in your blood or lymph liquid, phosphates pull it out of your bones.

Drinking sodas leads to lower levels of calcium in your body. You need calcium to help keep your colon clean. Calcium is a major mineral that your body uses to keep your body alkaline.

Sweets

Most sweets are made from highly processed ingredients and an abundance of sugar. Because sweets are unnatural food and contain no fiber, they contribute directly to constipation and should be avoided.

Sugars in sweets and in all other types of foods have a deteriorating effect on your body. Sugars in your body break down into many chemicals, one, which is alcohol. If you drink soda, the sugar in the soda supplies the body and brain with the alcohol ethanol.

Eat More Nutritious Food

Foods that activate peristalsis and have plenty of fiber
Fruits
- apricots apples cantaloupe avocado
- figs blackberries kiwi strawberries
- grapes cherries dates peaches
- raspberries pears pineapples oranges
- nectarines coconuts mangos papayas
- Persimmons plums prunes raisins
- cranberries elderberries currants gooseberries
- bananas

Vegetables

- collard greens kale dark green lettuce
- mustard greens spinach chard cabbage
- dandelion greens endives corn brussels sprouts
- eggplants asparagus Jerusalem artichoke,
- rhubarb rutabagas carrots celery cauliflower
- peas tomatoes turnips zucchini beets
- potatoes broccoli pumpkin corn squash
- bean sprouts green beans parsnip sweet potatoes
- radish peppers onions olives
- dulse chicory dandelion parsley watercress

Nuts, Beans, Grains

- sesame seeds walnuts pumpkin seeds pecans
- peanuts black walnuts almonds flaxseed
- lentils broad beans black beans
- pinto beans kidney beans chickpeas lima beans baked beans navy beans
- millet oats barley whole grains spinach pasta
- whole wheat pasta

Minimize cooking vegetable, since it reduces or breaks down the fiber.

Eat vegetables with skins when possible.

Broccoli has an anticancer compound called sulforaphane. This compound provides some protection against various types of cancer when used with 750 mg of N-acetyl-cysteine, NAC. The reason you want to take NAC is that it provides glutathione that works with sulforaphane to fight cancer. Add this vegetable and supplement to your diet to prevent colon cancer.

Eat More Fiber

If you are a cereal eater, this is a good time to eat more fiber. If not, then you can prepare a high fiber smoothie. Use more whole raw bran in your cereals. Or, you can grind up nuts and seed to add to your food.

Eating more fruits and vegetable will definitely give you more fiber.

Beans Stop Constipation

Beans are high in soluble and insoluble fiber. Eating them

helps to prevent constipation and contributes to lowering your cholesterol. Beans become viscous, a thick heavy fluid, as they pass through the intestines. This viscous fiber fluid is of benefit in your colon where it activates peristaltic action and promotes bowel movements.

Aside from lowering blood cholesterol and pressure, this viscous fiber in beans helps to decrease many types of colon diseases – cancer, colitis, and diverticulosis.

Most all types of beans have close to the same nutritional value. So eat the type you enjoy and gain their benefit.

One cup of cooked pinto or kidney beans has around 20 grams of fiber per cup. Lima and White beans have around 16 grams of fiber.

I don't recommend eating beans from cans. You have no control in their preparation. I recommend cooking beans in a crook pot by,

- Rinsing beans to remove dirt, tiny rocks, and bad beans
- Soaking beans for 2-4 hours in water
- Dumping the water from the soaked beans.
- Rinsing beans again but using distilled or reverse osmosis water
- Placing beans into the crook pot and cover with distilled water or reverse osmosis water
- Adding a couple of garlic cloves and onions
- Adding 2 to 3 capfuls of Eagle Brands Chili Powder

Turn crock-pot to low (not high) and cook beans for 8 hours or until beans are soft.

You can turn the crock-pot on low when you go to bed and in the morning you'll have cooked beans to eat for that day. Just make sure you have plenty of water covering your beans.

If you suffer from gout avoid beans, since they are high in purine.

Eat Good Oils

Good oils such as olive, flaxseed, evening primrose, black currant, and borage seed provide lubrication to the lining of your intestines and colon.
This lubrication of your colon and fecal matter is necessary for you to have regular bowel movements. Use these oils in place of mineral or castor oil.

Evening Primrose Oil - take 500 mg three times daily.

Omega-3 and Omega-6 are found in flax seeds and in fish, such as Alaskan salmon, tilapia, rainbow trout, cod and halibut. These are essential oils. Your body does not produce these oils, so they must be obtained from foods. Without omega-3 in your diet, you will be prone to constipation and many other painful diseases.

Fish

Do not eat fish for dinner. It is ok for lunch. Fish is hard to digest and you want to avoid foods that take to much time to digest during the evening.

Fish Oil

Fish oil contains omega-3 fatty acids, which are essential for good health. It has these fatty acids in the form of EPA, Eicosapentaenoic acid and DHA, docosahexaenoic acid.

Fatty acids help reduce inflammation through prostaglandin production. Prostaglandin's help reduces inflammation in your colon, which helps make your colon work better and reduces the possibility of constipation.

Use the enteric-coated fish oil capsules to reduce colon inflammation and to help reduce constipation.
Make sure when taking fish oil that is it is not fish liver oil. They are not the same food product. Fish liver oil can elevate blood sugar and cholesterol levels in some diabetics.

Fish oil can increase the rate of bleeding if you are using anticoagulant drugs such as warfarin, coumadin, or platelet inhibiting drugs - aspirin or ticlopidine.

Recommend dose of fish oil is 1000mg each day.

Flax Seeds

Flax seeds fall in the top 10 of healthy foods to live on. It contains a high-level of the omega-3 fatty acid that is essential for life. You cannot live without omega-3 fatty acid. Your diet must consist of a 3:1 or 4:1 ratio of omega-6 to omega 3. You must have 3 or 4 parts of omega-6 to 1 part of omega-3 in your diet.

Without this balance and with to much omega-6 fatty acid in your diet, you will be prone to illnesses related to,

Autoimmune diseases
Breast cancer
Cardiovascular diseases
Excessive blood clotting
Over drive of the immune system
Aside from all the benefits flax seeds provide, they also contain fiber and oils that will help prevent constipation. It contains 66% insoluble and 33% soluble fiber. Here is the nutritional breakdown for flax seeds.

- omega 3 - 41% to 57%

- omega 6 - 16%

- monounsaturated omega 9 - 18%

- saturated fat - 9%

- Fiber 28%

- Protein 20%

- Moisture 7%

- Ash 4%

The 57% omega-3 is considered plant source and differs from the omega-3 found in fish. Flax seed omega-3 is considered a short chain fatty acid and fish omega-3 is a long chain fatty acid.

Since your body only converts a small amount of flax seed omega-3 oil to EPA, you may want to also add fish oil to your diet, if you want the benefits of a higher level of EPA.

The recommendation for getting the proper amount of omega-3 into your diet is to eat fish 4 times a week and 1 ½ teaspoon of flax seeds. Few people meet this requirement.

So here is what you can do to get more omega-3 in your diet, so you can offset the bad effects too much omega-6 and reduce and prevent constipation.

Use 1-3 tablespoon of flax seed daily. Always grind these seeds with a coffee grinder. Then add them to your food.

- Add 1 teaspoon to your smoothie

- Add 1 teaspoon to your salad dressing

- Add 1 teaspoon to your cereal

Use flax seed without heating them. This preserves the nutritive value of this food and prevents its oxidation, which produces compounds that are not good for your health.

Garlic

Include raw garlic in your diet and in cooking. Garlic destroys harmful bacteria in your colon and penetrates your colon walls to loosen up accumulated waste.

Also, you can use aged garlic extract, which comes in a capsule. Aged garlic promotes the growth of good bacteria in your colon.

One added benefit of aged garlic is it absorbs heavy metals from the blood. Heavy metals are responsible for cell degradation.

Avoid using powdered garlic, since all its nutritive value has been lost during its heating process.

Lecithin For Nerve Protection

Lecithin is not talked about much, but it is a power nutrient that you should use frequently. Lecithin is needed to build the protective layer that surrounds the nerves that network throughout your body. Without this protective layer or with a worn layer, the information that is transmitted along these nerves suffers interference. This interference distorts the information that is sent from your brain into your body, causing malfunctions in various body systems.

The nerve network that surrounds your colon needs to be strong and stable, since it is constantly reacting to peristaltic activity.

Lecithin can be purchased in granules. Use it as an additive to all kinds of food preparations – smoothies, cereal, soups, salads, sauces, and gravies. It has very little taste.

Lecithin consists of 10-15% choline. Choline is used by the body to form acetylcholine. Acetylcholine is a neurotransmitter that is active in recalling memories.

Lecithin is one supplement that you must add to your eating pattern. It helps to break up fat into tiny bubbles that prevent fat from sticking to your artery walls.

Exercise

Exercise is necessary for reducing or minimizing constipation. Here is what exercising does for your colon and body,

- Tones and strengthen your colon muscles
- Eliminates blood toxins by sweating.
- Stimulates your cells to eliminate waste that is move into your lymphatic system
- Reduces tension and anxiety
- Stimulates your colon wall cell structure to increase its metabolic rate and thus improve its function.

Daily walks, after a meal, stimulate your colon for bowel movements. In addition, walking strengthens and tones your colon walls. This prevents your colon from becoming misshaped when you occasion become constipated.

Inactivity or lack of exercise will contribute to lack of colon muscle tone, which will contribute to constipation no matter what your age.

There are many good exercises that stimulate and strengthen your body. Any type of exercise will be of benefit for your health. When your colon is toxic, exercises activate the lymphatic system to remove that toxicity.

The lymphatic system removes waste and toxins from the liquid that surround your cells. So it is critical these toxins not be allowed to remain in your body long. If they do, then this is another form of constipation. Lymph nodes get plugged up with toxins, waste, and bacteria and as more waste and toxins are created they get backed up in the lymph liquid or vessels.

Feed the Good Bacteria

The good bacteria, in your colon, are known by many names – good bacteria, micro flora, and probiotics. This bacterium is necessary for good colon and body health. The main bacteria in your colon are:

- Lactobacillus acidophilus
- Bifidobacterium bifidum
- Lactobacillus salivarius
- Bifidobacterium infantis
- Streptococcus faecium

When buying probiotics, buy a mixture of these bacteria. In some products, you will find added Fructo-oligosccharides, FOS, which helps to feed the good bacteria and promote their survival.

Cultured yogurt is a good way to get additional good bacteria into your colon. The best way to eat it is in-between meals. The best yogurt to eat is goat milk yogurt. It costs a bit more, but it is worth the health benefits you get from it.

Look for yogurt that says the bacteria culture was added after pasteurization. If the yogurt was pasteurized after the bacteria culture was added, the good bacteria would have been destroyed.

Eat yogurt at least 3 times a week. You can add flax seed oil, berries, raisins, flax seed grounds, or other toppings that promote bowel movements.

The best way to get probiotics or good bacteria into your colon is to take a supplement, liquid or pill, between meals with distilled water. When probiotics are taken with food, food increases the stomach acid, which destroys the probiotic supplement.

Eating cultured vegetables is another way to get probiotics or good bacteria. Some flora-enhanced foods are:

- Sauerkraut
- Yogurt
- Kefir
- Miso
- Micro alga

5: Minerals And Nutrients For Constipation

Taking A Good Mineral Supplement

To maintain a strong and active colon, you need to take a good mineral supplement, which contain plenty of sodium, magnesium, calcium, and potassium. In addition, you need to get these minerals from the food you eat. Food has a balance of these minerals and nutrient you need to build your colon and other parts of your body.

Potassium

Potassium is needed to keep your colon walls working properly and for keeping them free of acid, which attracts disease. It helps to dislodge colon wastes that accumulate along your colon walls.

Potassium tastes bitter so most of the foods that are bitter contain potassium, especially herbal teas. Best foods to eat for high levels of potassium are:

- Cucumbers
- Bitter greens
- Lentils
- Almonds
- Oatmeal
- Potato skins
- German prunes
- American prunes
- Peaches
- Gooseberries
- Romaine lettuce
- Figs

- Carrots
- apples
- apple cider vinegar
- apricots
- bananas
- beans
- blueberries
- goat milk
- grapes
- pears
- raisins
- tomatoes
- sesame seeds
- beets and prunes

Prepare A Miracle Mineral Salad

Prepare a green salad like this,

- Cut up romaine or dark green lettuce

- Cut up carrots and cucumbers

- chopped garlic cloves

- chopped onions

- 2-3 tablespoons of apple cider vinegar

- 2 tablespoons of olive oil

- 1 tablespoon of flax seed oil

- 1 tablespoon of lecithin

- hard-boiled eggs.

The allicin in the garlic is invigorated by the minerals in the onion and penetrates the large intestine wall to stimulate it.

The fiber, in the vegetables helps to scrub the intestinal walls. The vinegar boosts enzymatic action of the allicin and the allicin stimulates peristaltic movement. The oils helps to lubricate the stools and colon walls. Lecithin breaks down oil into fine drops, which are absorbed quickly through the intestinal walls.

This is a natural way to dissolve accumulated toxic wastes on your colon walls and to eliminate them.

Here is a garlic salad helps keep your intestinal walls clean.

- juice to two cloves of garlic
- 2 tablespoon of flaxseed oil
- 3 tablespoons of olive oil
- 1 tablespoon of balsamic vinegar
- 2 tablespoons of apple cider vinegar
- ground up flax or sunflower seeds
- one tablespoon of bran

You can add other vegetables you like to this salad.

Digestive enzymes

Digestive enzymes help you digest and absorb your food and supplements.   To digest different types of food, your body produces different enzymes such as,

- Protease – for digesting protein
- Lactase – for digesting lactose a protein in milk
- Amylase – for digesting carbohydrate
- Pepsin – for digesting protein

Do not use digestive enzymes if you have ulcers.

Amylase starts carbohydrate digestion in your mouth. The longer you chew your food, which is a healthy practice, the better digested your food will be. Your stomach will not have to work as hard and less undigested food will reach your colon.

Raw fruits and vegetables have their own digestive enzymes, which help to digest themselves. When fruits or vegetables are heated above 120 F, their enzymes are destroyed and no longer available to your body. When this happens, your body has to create these enzymes to digest this cooked food. This takes energy and enzymes away from within your body that could be used elsewhere to do more important work.

When you eat cooked food, processed and packaged food, you use excessive digestive enzymes. Sometimes not all your food is digested properly, and these undigested remains move into your colon where they create gas, toxic material, which weakens your colon walls.

Pregnant

If you are pregnant, here is a way to start or assist your bowel movement. When sitting on the toilet, raise your legs to the same level of the toilet seat by placing your legs on a chair. Lean back slightly and place your arms above your head. You can also try moving left and right to move or stretch the sigmoid and rectum to help produce a bowel movement.

High Fiber Breakfasts

Oatmeal Cereal

Use oatmeal that takes 5-6 minutes to cook. This type of oatmeal has had a minimum of processing. Do not use the instant oatmeal that takes one minute to cook.

Cook oatmeal with distilled water for 5-6 minutes.
Add a heaping tablespoon of bran with the oatmeal you put into the boiling water.

Cut a small apple into tiny pieces and add them and raisins to the oatmeal after it has boiled for a couple of minutes about one minute before you pull the oatmeal off the stove, add a tablespoon of granular lecithin.

You can add 1/2 banana, which is not too ripe. The banana will sweeten up your oatmeal. The riper the banana the higher the banana will be in sugar. Add 1 tablespoon of edible-grade dairy whey.

After the oatmeal is cooked, add a little apple juice, rice dream, or almond milk to thin it down and sweeten slightly. If you like, you can add a bit of honey.

Other things you can add to this breakfast are:

- Grounded flax seeds, but add them after the oatmeal has cooled a little.
- A small amount of pure maple syrup
- 1/8 teaspoon of cinnamon
- A date or two instead of raisins

Anti-Oxidant Breakfast Fruit Salad

One of the most important health discoveries in the past decades is the importance of antioxidants. They are capable of neutralizing free radicals in our body. It is free radicals, which you take in from the air and food that destroy your cell's ability to function normally. This holds true for our colon cells, which eventually leads to poor colon function.

Here is a fruit salad that can provide you with a high-level of antioxidants.

- 1 orange or grapefruit peeled and sliced
- 1 small mango (the small yellow ones)
- 1 banana
- 1 kiwi
- 1 apple sliced
- a small amount of fresh pineapple
- some strawberries
- some blueberries and red grapes.

6: Natural Juices For Constipation Remedies

Organic Juices

Organic fresh made juices have cleansing and laxative action. These juices contain loads of mineral, bioflavonoids, vitamins, enzymes, antioxidants, and other nutrients. Citric fruits have citric acid and the more tart they are the more acid they have.

Fresh juice is a fast way to get all types of nutrients into your blood quickly. As juice nutrients get into your blood, they suck out toxins and build up tissues. In your colon, they destroy bacteria, feed wall tissue, pull out toxins, and activate peristaltic action.

Even though juices provide helpful action throughout the body, it is best to limit their use and drink them in larger quantities, only when trying to accomplish certain health benefits. Always use fresh or organic juices when possible.

When juicing fruits and vegetables, the more fiber that is left with the juice the better results you will get with your constipation.

It is always best to use fresh juices, but as a last resort using packaged juices will be better than not drinking anything. And, buy your juices in glass containers, if you can.

Drink your juices between meals and not during your meals. When you do this you will gain the benefit of the peristaltic action these juices provide. You should wait about 1 to 1 1/2 after meals before drinking juices or eating fruit.

Apples and Apple Juice

Apples are good for eliminating constipation because they are high in pectin, a soluble fiber, have many minerals, and contain Sorbitol - a natural sugar, which stimulates peristaltic action. Pectin helps to detoxify the intestines and promote regular bowel movements.

The fiber in apples adds weight and bulk to your fecal matter. It helps draw water from your colon chamber into the fecal matter. This keeps the stools from becoming hard and difficult to move through your colon.

Apples are one of best fruits to eat because they are high in minerals, which provide alkaline electrolytes to your body. What this does is neutralize acids that are created during illness, anxiety, anger, exercising, breathing pollution, and improper eating. Body acids are a major reason we get deadly diseases as we age.

Make eating apples or drinking fresh apple juice a daily habit. They are also effective in liver and gallbladder problems.

Here's what to do.

Use crisp and hard apples, such as granny smith, fuji, or gala for juicing.

Drink three glasses of apple juice each day, morning, noon, and evening. In combination with drinking fresh apple juice, eat 3-4 apples each day to get fiber.

One-day apple and apple juice fast

You can also do a one-day apple and apple juice fast by,
Eat 3-4 apples during the day. Drink apples juice every two hours. Don't eat anything until the next morning.

Apple Juice, Figs and Raisins

Here's another recipe using apple juice. Use it the first thing in the morning before breakfast.

In a blender, put in a cup of fresh apple juice. Add equal amounts of dry or fresh figs and raisins. Choose how many figs and raisins to use. You will need to experiment a little. Get a consistency that is not too thick. Add a little more apple juice if needed.

Boysenberry

Boysenberry juice has a gentle natural laxative action on your bowel. When your constipation is mild, this juice will help move things in your colon.

Blackberries

Mix ½ cup of distilled water and ½ cup of blackberry juice. Drink this first thing in the morning or between meals to promote peristaltic movement. Drink this often and it will make you regular.

Cherries

Cherries are high in antioxidants, fiber, potassium, and many other minerals, which are effective in neutralizing body acids. Cherries contain vitamins B-1, B-2, folic acid and niacin.

Cherries have strong laxative effects and can start peristaltic action. Eat fresh cherries throughout the day or drink three 8 oz glasses of cherry juice during the day. Buy cherry juice in glass container.

Elderberry Juice

Elderberry juice can be used to help reduce the symptoms of

colds, flu, and diabetes. It also helps to relieve constipation, diarrhea, and hemorrhoids. Drink 1–2 glasses each day. Increase the quantity if necessary

Citrus Juices

Citrus juices are an excellent way to stimulate your colon and other parts of the body. Since your colon is less active at night, drink these juices as soon as you awaken and get up. This can stimulate strong peristaltic action and promote a bowel movement.

Lemons

Lemons are filled with minerals, especially potassium, vitamin C, and bioflavonoids. They have a cleansing action for the entire body. They help you get rid of mucus inside the body and have a cleansing effect on your blood.

Fresh lemon juice is the king of fruit juices. It contains citric acid, which acts in the body in a way no other juice does. First it acts on the liver to build up its enzymes, so it can detoxify toxins in the blood. Then it combines with calcium to form a soluble chemical that makes it effective in removing kidney and pancreatic stones. This soluble chemical also prevents plaque buildup along artery walls, and other calcium deposits that occur in your body.

When the liver, gallbladder, and pancreas are not working right, food digestion is affected. This in turn will create constipation.

Use lemons moderately since they break up oils during digestion and in your body, making oils less available to your cells and joints.

If you have lemon allergies or ulcers then you should avoid lemon juice. If you have arthritis, lemons are not a good choice.

Here's what to do:

Squeeze one lemon into a glass of warm distilled water. Drink it first thing when you wake up. Don't drink or eat anything for at least 1/2 hour.

You can use a citrus press to juice the lemon or just squeeze it to get the juice out.

7: Fruits That Help With Constipation

Fruits The Perfect Food

Fruits are made by nature and are a perfect food. They contain the right balance of nutrients with distilled water. You gain enormous benefits from eating fruits, especially if you eat the outer skin. They should be eaten without cooking. They are easy to digest and absorb and do not stress your colon.

Fruits contain fiber, which help to cleanse your colon and prevent constipation. Most fruits help provide the body with minerals that help the body reduce acid as it is created. And most important of all, fruits help cleanse the body of mucus slime that accumulates throughout the body.

Fruits do not leave any slime residue in the body when eaten, except when they have pesticides and preservatives in their outer skin. They do not ferment or putrefy in your colon, as do processed foods, dairy products and meats.

Choose your fruits carefully. They should be eaten when fully ripe. Do not eat them, if they are under ripe or overripe. In the under ripe condition, they may be acidic, and in the overripe condition they may contain more natural sugar.

Fruits, vegetables, and grains contain fructooligosaccharides, FOS. It is this compound that helps to feed the good bacteria in your colon. Without an adequate supply of FOS, good bacteria will dwindle and bad bacteria will flourish.

Here is a list of fruits that will help you eliminate constipation. Eat them for breakfast or between meals.

Bananas

Bananas are rich in potassium. They assist in healing open wounds in the interior body membranes. They are helpful in stopping diarrhea and at the same time in promoting bowel movements.

Eat two bananas on an empty stomach followed by a glass of distilled water. After your constipation is cleared, eat only one banana each day.

Blue berries

Blue berries can act as a laxative for some people despite its use to stop diarrhea. These berries have the chemical anthocyanosides that can kill bacteria and viruses.

Blueberries are also good for reducing inflammation. This makes them good for inflammations that occur all along the gastrointestinal tract.

Boysenberries

Boysenberry juice has a gentle natural laxative action on your bowel. When your constipation is not extra serious, this juice will help move things in your colon.

Cantaloupe

Cantaloupe is one of the best fruits you can eat. It contains many minerals and has Vitamin A and C. It is high in potassium. It has plenty of fiber and is useful for constipation.

Cherries

Cherries are high in potassium, fiber, and many other minerals, which are effective in neutralizing body acid. They contain vitamins B-1, B-2, folic acid and niacin.

Cherries have excellent laxative effect and can start peristaltic action.

Eat fresh cherries throughout the day or drink 3 glasses, 8 oz, of cherry juice during the day. Buy cherry juice in glass containers.

Dried cherries can also be used except they can be expensive.

Figs and Dates

Figs are high in fiber and can provide a gentle action on your colon, when you have been constipated. This action can take about 24 hours before it takes place.

The use of figs and dates combined can have a stronger action on your colon.

Grapes

Grapes have good laxative action. Eat 1-2 lbs of grapes though out the day. Reduce the amount of food you eat during the day. Eat more vegetables and other fruits. Reduce the amount of processed foods you eat.

Grapes are high in vitamins and minerals. They have good fiber content and are especially high in manganese.

Since they are high in sugar, bugs are attracted to them. This causes farmers to spray them with pesticides. Try to find them at the farmer's market as organic or not sprayed.

Papaya

Papaya is well known for its enzyme papain, which helps digest protein. Its minerals help reduce cell waste and eliminate stomach and colon mucus.

Persimmon

Eat 2-3 persimmons each day, if they are available. They help to keep you regular.

Plums

Fresh plums are filled with minerals and have a mild laxative effect. They can relieve gas and have a cleansing effect on your intestines.

Prunes

Prunes are dried plums. Eat both for their natural laxative effect.

Prunes are more effective than plums for constipation. Buy a bag of dried prunes and eat them throughout the day. Aside from this laxative effect, prunes are high in iron.

Raspberries

Raspberries are high in vitamins A and C. They are high in magnesium, calcium, and iron. They are helpful in clearing constipation.

8: Vegetables To Use For Constipation

The benefits of Vegetables

Juices are absorbed quickly into your bloodstream. As a result, your cells are provided quickly with nutrients that feed them and that wash away waste. Juices give you the opportunity to get quick relief from various body conditions such as constipation. Juices move into your colon quickly to cleanse it and to activate peristaltic action.

Eating and drinking vegetables and their juices provide you with minerals and nutrients that build your blood, tissue, bones, and cells. It is minerals that build every part of your body. It is minerals that keep your body's pH at the required level. It is minerals that keep your body alkaline by neutralizing body acids.

It is minerals that build your colon wall tissues and cells, so your colon can perform those activities that prevent constipation.

So, let's look at which vegetables and vegetable juices can help you end constipation.

Keep in mind that some natural recipes for clearing constipation require drinking vegetable juices that are bitter or have a strong taste. As you will find, some of the vegetable juices taste good and some don't. Remember you are dealing with a condition that needs clearing and that what you drink for this is and not for pleasure.

As you drink some of these vegetable juices, you may find that you like certain ones and these can become your regular daily or weekly drink.

Carrot Juice

Carrot juices contain certain oils that work on the mucus membranes of the stomach and colon. This helps with digestion and starts your bowels functioning properly. Carrots are high in fiber and beta-carotene, an antioxidant, which the body converts to vitamin A. Carrots can make your stools softer and larger.

Why are larger stools better? Because larger stools dilute toxins, exposure fewer toxins to colon walls, and press against colon walls to promote peristaltic action.

Drink carrot juice twice daily, once in the morning and in the evening before bedtime.

You can drink more carrot juice if you like. Its action on the body produces enormous benefits, since it contains a good number of vitamins and minerals – B, C, D, E, K, carotene, sodium, and potassium. These nutrients help to clean out your colon and speed up fecal matter movement.

As you increase the carrot juice you drink, chances are you will feel a little uncomfortable. This happens when carrot juice reaches your intestines and colon and begins stirring up the toxic layers and materials in that area. This feeling will pass and is nothing to worry about.

If you are pregnant, drink carrot juice daily to build up your breast milk and to provide your baby with the nutrients that it needs.

Carrot Juice, Carrots and Celery

An effective way to clear constipation is to combine vegetables that are high in fiber with those that have laxative effects.

Celery is high in fiber, potassium, sodium, and many other minerals. It can reduces inflammation and protect against cancer.

Celery has a chemical call polyacetylene, which reduces prostaglandins that cause inflammation.

Celery has a calming effect on the nervous system. If you have been using laxatives, which have overworked your colon nerves, celery will help to relax these nerves and give them a rest.

Adding carrot juice to celery juice provides an even better nutritional drink. This drink will help to restore nerve function in your colon and improve its health.

Celery has the highest content of organic sodium. This sodium is used throughout the body as lymph saline liquid allowing cells to work and live properly. This sodium will reduce the acid accumulation that occurs in the lymph liquid.

Celery is also beneficial for the stomach. The stomach lining is filled with sodium and this sodium necessary to prevent ulcers.

Here's what to do,

Eat carrots and celery during the day and for your salads; drink a glass of carrot juice in the morning and one in afternoon. By eating slightly steamed carrots you can increase the carotene available from the carrot by up to 4 times. However, by cooking carrots, you destroy the enzymes that will help you to digest them quickly and completely.

Boost your carrot juice by juicing with it a few stalks of celery, which includes the leaves. The leaves have more nutrients than the stalk and are part of the nutritional value of the celery.

Tomato, Carrot, Celery Drink

Here's a drink you can take in the afternoon to activate a bowel movement.

With a juicer, juice some tomatoes, carrots, and celery. By experimenting, you can discover the amount of each vegetable to use according to your taste. Mostly likely you will want equal amounts of tomatoes and carrots and you will want to add a few stalks of celery including the leaves.

Now, let's add a few more items to give your drink more pushing power. Squeeze in a small amount of garlic, onion, and radish.

While juicing your carrots, juice a small bunch of spinach or parsley.

Drink 1 to 1 ½ cups in the morning.

Carrots, Cabbage and Raisins

Because carrots contain fiber, they help to form a good stool and promote peristaltic action. By combining carrots with cabbage and raisins, you can create an even more powerful food that will help in relieving constipation. Combine the following vegetables to form an evening salad:

- Chopped carrots
- Shredded cabbage (raw or slightly steamed)
- Romaine lettuce
- Cauliflower
- Cucumbers

- A handful raisins
- Sprinkle a tablespoon of grounded flax seeds
- Mix in 1 – 2 tablespoons of olive oil
- Mix in 2 tablespoons of apple cider vinegar
- One tablespoon of lecithin granules

Eat this salad once or twice a day for three days. After that you should continue to eat a vegetable salad for lunch or dinner.

Carrot and Spinach Juice

Combine 10 oz of carrot and 6 oz of spinach juice. Drink two pints daily. Both these vegetables have nutrients to help relieve your constipation.

Cucumber

Cucumbers are good for preventing constipation. But they can be used in the carrot-spinach juice or the apple-spinach juice. Cucumbers make these juices more powerful. Use only about ¼ - ½ of a cucumber when adding it to these juices. You can experiment with how much cucumber you want to add.

Cucumbers are a natural diuretic and help to dissolve kidney stones.

Because they are high in potassium, they help to promote the flexibility of colon cells. This helps to keep your colon working, as it should.

9: Herbal Natural Constipation Remedies

Herbal Remedies

Herbal laxatives help to promote bowel movements and relieve constipation. They remove food and toxic build up along your colon walls. When used in combinations, more than one herb, herbs provide nutrients and substances that help to feed and tone your colon walls and at the same time move fecal matter out through the rectum.

Strong Herbal Laxatives

Herbal laxatives can be weak, moderate, or strong. Strong laxatives are called cathartics or purgatives and are used when you have a severe case of constipation.

The strong herbs are Aloe Vera, Buckthorn, Cascara Sagrada, Chinese Rhubarb and Senna. They work by stimulating or irritating your colon wall nerves to promote a strong peristaltic movement.

Care must be taken when using strong laxatives, since they have an irritating effect on your colon walls and sometimes can be painful and griping. As with drugstore laxatives, these strong herbs can create a lazy colon requiring you to use them over and over to have a bowel movement.

You will find some herbs mixed in with drugstore laxatives.

Weak and Moderate Herbal Laxatives

The best herbal laxatives to use are those that promote digestive juice secretions, which activate a bowel movement.

Moderate herbal laxatives are herbs like licorice, Wahoo, Yellow Dock, Balmony, Barberry, Dandelion Root, flax seeds, and psyllium seeds.

Some herbal combinations are listed below that combine weak, moderate, and strong herbal laxatives. These combinations provide the benefits of both herbs and reduce the strong effects of the individual herbs.

Preparing Herbal Teas

When preparing an herbal tea, called an infusion, it is best to use a glass, porcelain-lined or stainless steel pot with a cover. Boil distilled water, then, remove the pot from the stove. Do not use a microwave to heat your water. Microwaves change the electrical characteristics of water.

Place the herbs into hot water and stir. Cover the pot and let it sit for 5-30 minutes. The longer herbs sit in the water the stronger the tea becomes. After the tea cools a bit, strain it, and it is ready to drink. If the tea is too bitter for you, you can add a touch of honey.

Use one teaspoon to one tablespoon of mixed herbs to 1 ¼ cup of distilled water.

If you are pregnant, do not use any of herbs listed in this chapter, since they are designed to promote contractions in your colon and surrounding areas.

Children's Herbal Dosage

When giving children herbal products use more care.
Give a reduced amount based on the adult dosage.

Children's Age and Dose

- 10-14 years use 1/2 adult herbal dose

- 6-10 years use 1/3 adult herbal dose
- 2-6 years use 1/4 adult herbal dose

Licorice Root

Licorice root has a mild laxative effect. It is good for ulcers and inhibits the growth of harmful viruses. It has high-sugar content, so diabetics should use it with caution.

Licorice root stimulates the endocrine system to use up potassium and sodium at a faster rate. So it would be wise to use Alkalife in your drinking water, when using licorice, to add sodium and potassium back into your system.

Licorice may also lower testosterone level in men. Men suffering from impotence, infertility may want to avoid this herb.

Licorice makes your body hold water. Do not use Licorice, if you have high blood pressure, are pregnant, or use corticosteroid drugs. Licorice root may increase the side effects of these drugs.

If using digoxin, or diuretic drugs do not use licorice root since it pushes potassium out in the urine.

Deglycrrhizinated, DGL, may be O.K. to use with these drug, but check with your doctor to make sure.

Prepare 1 cup of tea, using one tablespoon of licorice root. Drink 3 times each day.

Anise seed tea

Anise seeds produce a tea that can improve your digestion, which helps to reduce constipation. Anise seed tea is also good for improving memory, brain activity, and overall body health.

Take two tablespoons of anise seeds and put them into a coffee grinder. Press the start button for 2-3 second just to break up the seed lightly.

Make a tea with these seed as follows:

Boil 1 ½ cup of distilled water in a glass pot. Pull the pot off the stove and put the seeds into the water and cover the pot. Let the seeds sit in water for 10-15 minutes to make a good strong tea.

Drink one cup of this tea first thing in the morning.

Alfalfa Tea

Alfalfa helps to relieve constipation. It is rich in fiber, minerals, and chlorophyll. It is helpful in improving gastrointestinal function.

Warfarin and alfalfa interaction – Alfalfa is a high source of vitamin K, which helps blood to clot. This has the opposite of effect of the drug Warfarin, which helps to thin the blood to avoid clotting. If you are under a doctor's care and using Warfarin consult your doctor before using Alfalfa herb.

Alfalfa has many minerals, so it is considered an alkalizing food. It contains C, E, K, and B vitamins making it one of the best herbs for building the body back to health.

Since alfalfa helps reduce infections, it is useful in infections that occur in your colon and throughout your body.

Prepare a cup of tea by using a tablespoon of alfalfa leaves in boiling water. Let it sit for 10 –15 minutes off the stove. This tea has a strong grassy taste and you may want to add a bit of honey or lemon to reduce its strong taste.

Elderflower

Drink a tea of elderflower daily to relieve constipation

Chickweed

Drink 1 cup of chickweed every 3 hours and do this until you have a bowel movement.

Chinese Rhubarb

Chinese rhubarb, rhubarb, and turkey rhubarb has been used for many decades to relieve constipation in China. It has a strong purgative action – it encourages strong laxative stimulation. It should be combined with other herbs, which reduces its purgative strength.

Pregnant women should not use Rhubarb.

Rhubarb, Ginger, licorice Infusion

- For severe constipation, prepare an infusion of,
- 1 teaspoon of rhubarb powder
- ¼ teaspoon of ginger root
- ¼ teaspoon of licorice root
- Drink 1/2 cup of this infusion and over a few days increase it to a cup.

Chlorophyll

Chlorophyll is the green substance that occurs in all plants and is one of the most helpful substances you can add to your diet. It helps to strengthen and thicken your colon cell walls. It inhibits the growth of disease producing pathogenic bacteria and feeds the good bacteria.

It detoxifies the cells in your body and colon, which houses an unbelievable amount of toxic matter.

Chlorophyll will help to get your bowels moving by improving your colon function. Use chlorophyll with any of the other methods you use to clear your constipation.

Take 2 capsules of chlorophyll just before meals

The way that I use chlorophyll is by combining 1-2 oz. liquid chlorophyll, juice of one lemon, and 8 oz. of distilled water, first thing in the morning. This combination sits really well in my stomach, and I have never had an upset stomach from this drink.

You can also add one or two tablespoons of chlorophyll to a glass of one-half orange and one-half grapefruit juice. With this mixture, you will not taste the chlorophyll much.

Chlorophyll is considered safe for pregnant and lactating women.

Triphala

Here is a well-known and popular India Ayurvedic herbal product that is available on the Internet and perhaps in some India food stores.

It is called Triphala. It is effective as a laxative and also has many other benefits such as:

- Improves liver function and digestion
- Reduces high blood pressure and serum cholesterol

Triphala comes from 3 fruits tree – Harada, Amla, and Bihara.

Harada is used to treat chronic and acute constipation and anxiety.

Amla, known for its high vitamin C content and is used to treat body imbalances in the liver, stomach, and intestines. It also fights infections throughout the body.

Bihara is used to balance and purify excess mucus in the body and especially in the intestines and colon.

Use Triphala for two – three weeks and longer if necessary. This is one combination that you can use for 2-3 months at a time.

Mix ½ teaspoon of Triphala powder with 8 oz of warm water and drink just before bedtime.

Or, Take 2 capsules in the morning and 2 capsules just before you go to bed.

Senna Tea

You can also prepare senna tea as follows:

Buy some senna tea at a health food. Place a tea bag into 1 ½ cups of distilled water and steep. Then, add the peel of a whole red potato. Also, add a couple slices of potato meat. Add to this, a teaspoon of wheat or oat bran and flax seed.

Simmer this combination, strain it and drink the liquid. This will help some of the more difficult cases of constipation. Remember the longer you simmer this combination the stronger the tea will be.

Start with a 5-10 minutes and then work up to 15-20 minutes, but you need to experiment with the time.

When you drink senna tea, drink only 2-3 oz. at a time and

drink it only after it has cooled down. It has less of a cramping action when you drink it cold.

Senna Tea with Mint

Here is another senna tea you can prepare.

- 1 teaspoon of senna tea leaves
- ½ teaspoon of peppermint leaves.

Boil 8 oz. of distilled water, turn the heat off, and stir in the herbs. Turn the heat off and cover the glass container. Let tea simmer for 3-10 minutes. Add honey and/or vitamin C to improve taste, if you have it.

Look for formulas that have a small amount, 1/10 of a part, of fennel, anise, or ginger to reduce any cramping that might occur with senna. You can add these amounts to the teas listed above.

Do not drink senna tea or capsule if you have any type of colon disease, stomach pain, diarrhea, or are pregnant.

Senna Pods are milder than the leaves, since the do not contain resin. It is the resin in the senna leaves that causes griping in your colon.

If available, use around 8 pods. Heat some distilled water. Place the pods into the water for 5-10 minutes. Strain the tea and add 3-4 dried prunes or chopped prunes. Let cool and eat the prunes during the day or drink and eat a few prunes just before you go to bed. Drink only a couple ounces of the senna liquid at one time. If cramping or griping occurs, reduce the amount of tea you drink.

10: Minerals And Vitamins For Constipation

Minerals

Minerals help the body produce energy and build bones, blood and cells. They are found in the blood and lymph liquid and cell walls.

They help in nerve transmission and muscle contractions in your colon. Minerals are used with vitamins and other nutrients to form compounds that are essential for your body's health.

Your body cannot create minerals so you have to get them from the food you eat or through supplements.

Vitamins

Vitamins do not provide energy for the body, they are not found in your tissue, and they do not build cells. They help in converting the food you eat over to nutrients that your body can use. This means they help enzymes break down your food - protein, fat, and carbohydrates. Your body can make only a few vitamins.

Mineral and Vitamin Supplements

The various minerals and vitamins recommended here can be taken individually or as a multi-mineral complex or as a vitamin complex. Avoid a supplement that contains both vitamins and minerals. There is some loss in the effectiveness of individual vitamins and minerals when they are combined in multiform. When a lot of nutrients are put into a pill, the amount of each nutrient becomes less, making the pill ineffective. Use capsules for best results because capsules are filled with powder.

Capsules dissolve quickly and so does the powder.

Some hard, tablet supplements may not dissolve completely in your stomach or intestines and flow into your colon and out your rectum. It is estimated that when you use a hard tablet, you only absorb around 15 – 20% of its value.

Minerals In Fruits and Vegetables

Minerals in produce are the best minerals to take. These minerals are in the form that nature created and is exactly what the body needs. They are electo-magnetically charged and have a life force that is provided by the plant. This life force quickly decreases after the fruit or vegetable has been picked.

Therefore, it is always recommended to eat fruits or vegetable soon after they have been picked and not to cook them.

You can get electrolytic minerals in liquid form on the Internet. If you decide not to use them, use chelated minerals. Chelated minerals are attached to amino acids making them magnetic, which allow them to flow right through the intestinal walls, without having to be digested.

Look for minerals such as,

- Calcium aspartate
- Calcium gluconate
- Calcium Citrate

Mineral Absorption

Most minerals are absorbed in the last part of the small intestine and the beginning of the large intestine, your colon. When your colon walls collect layer upon layer of waste, it affects absorption of the minerals you consume. When this happens, your body will be deficient in minerals and your appetite will be larger than normal.

Brewer's Yeast

Brewer's Yeast contains all B vitamins, except B12. It also contains many vitamins, minerals and is high in amino acids. Brewer's yeast can help to ease, reduce, or clear your constipation. If you can handle the taste, add it to your juices, morning and night.

When you first use brewer's yeast, it will create gas in your colon. Brewer's yeast provides food to your good bacteria in your colon, increasing its count. This increase in good bacteria activates a battle between the good and bad bacteria creating gas as a by-product.

Keep using brewer's yeast until the gas stops. This many take a few weeks but you are doing one of the best things you can do for your health – increasing good bacteria and reducing bad bacteria.

You can improve the benefits of using brewer's yeast by eating cultured yogurt or supplementing with good bacteria between meals. You want to take good bacteria supplements between meals, so your stomach acid does not increase and destroy the bacteria.

If you have gout or are taking monoamine oxidase inhibitors do not take brewers yeast.

MSM

MSM stands for methyl sulfonyl methane. MSM is organic

sulfur.

It provides many benefits in the body and is widely used as an anti- inflammatory and is especially useful for arthritis pain. MSM is used in all body cells and tissue including joint tissue.

MSM in your colon stops or blocks the activity of cholinesterase (ko-li-nes-ter-ace.)

What Is cholinesterase?

Your nervous system is composed of a network of nerve cells, which start at the brain and end on all parts of your body. It is nerves that direct muscle contraction or expansion. After the muscle completes its movement, an enzyme cholinesterase is released, which stops the muscle movement. Without this enzyme, the muscle would continue to move nonstop.

MSM is useful in clearing up constipation. When I have used MSM, up to 6000 - 8000mg each day, I have experienced up to 3-4 bowel movements each day. As MSM blocks the activity of cholinesterase, it allows more peristaltic action to occur in your colon. This results in more bowel movements.

Using 2000-4000mg of MSM, should produce one to two bowel movements each day. Of course, for each person the amount will be different.

The action that MSM has in the colon is useful for older adults, who have less nerve signals for peristalsis. Cholinesterase stops the few peristalsis signals older people have, thus creating constipation.

Vitamins

The following vitamins help in normalizing and clearing constipation:

Vitamin A

Vitamin A should never be taken by itself. It should be used with other vitamins or taken with food or with fruit snacks.
When taken alone, Vitamin A will putrefy in your colon creating toxic chemicals that may get into your blood.

Vitamin A helps to protect your mucous membrane along the gastrointestinal tract from bacterial attacks. It is also effective in reducing kidney and gallbladder stones.
Vitamin A is essential for a healthy liver. For some individuals, taking vitamin A daily would eliminate constipation.

Vitamin A is an important vitamin, which helps to improve your immunity. Since your colon is an important part of your immune system, it is recommended you eat those foods that are high in Vitamin A or to use a Vitamin A supplement. Vitamin A will strengthen your colon.

Vitamin A also helps you absorb protein in your small intestine. Any protein that is not absorbed will move into your colon undigested. In this form and in your colon, this protein decays producing highly toxic material that can cause serious illness over time.

If you are pregnant or planning to get pregnant, do not take more than 5000 IU each day to avoid birth defects. Make sure you talk to your doctor on how much vitamin A to take.

If you have any liver disease, consult your doctor before taking vitamin A.

Foods high in vitamin A are,

Green leaf vegetables, carrots, eggs, yellow vegetables, butter, liver, cabbage, prunes, celery, parsley, spinach, kale, cheese, tomatoes.

B-Vitamins

B-vitamins are needed to feed your colon wall nerves so they can flex and move naturally. Without these vitamins your colon walls cannot move in a natural rhythm.

Eat less sugar and sweets, since these foods use up B-vitamins when being digested.

Take Thiamine (B1) 100-300 mg each day, since it helps to correct constipation by stimulating peristalsis.

Inositol – Helps stimulate your colon walls. Inadequate inositol can be associated with constipation. Drinking too much coffee reduces inositol from the body. Use 100 – 300 mg each day

Folic Acid - If you have constipation and have leg cramps, you may need folic acid. In this case take 400-800 IU of folic acid each day.

Pantothenic acid - 5mg to 500mg before bed improves the health of your colon.

Vitamin C

Taking Vitamin C will help to keep you regular. It is a gentle laxative when taken in high doses. When you become constipated, increase your use of Vitamin C. Add 500 mg each day until you reach 7000 mg. At some point, you may experience diarrhea. When this happens, just back off on the dose by 500 mg. When your constipation is cleared go back to your maintenance dose.

Vitamin C in doses greater than 500 mg is not recommended if you have kidney stone, liver disease, or gout.

Vitamin C may increase your absorption of Aluminum, if you

are taking antacids. Take vitamin C two hours before taking antacids, to prevent this problem.

Recommend vitamin C dose is 2500 – 3500 mg each day taken with meals. Pregnant women can take up to 500 mg each day.

Calcium

In your colon, calcium combines with excess bile and decaying fat to form a harmless insoluble soap, which is excreted with your stool. This helps to keep your colon clean.
Most Nutritionists recommend you take 1000 - 1500mg daily of Calcium. Because Calcium can cause constipation, it is necessary to take 500 – 1000mg of magnesium at the same time you take Calcium. Space out your intake of calcium over the day.

Take only 400 to 600mg each time. Also take some time-out when taking calcium and other vitamin supplements. In a month, take 2-3 Sundays or Saturdays off from taking vitamins.

Avoid taking calcium carbonate, which will reduce the times you will have a bowel movement. Avoid, also, taking calcium when eating foods that contain oxalates phosphates, or phytates – cooked spinach or rhubarb. They tie up calcium and are excreted with the fecal matter.

If you have cancer, kidney disease, irregular heartbeat, or hyperparathyroidism consult your doctor before using calcium supplements.

If you are taking a thyroid hormones, beta - blockers, calcium-channel blockers, or antibiotics, calcium supplements can interfere with adsorption of these drugs.

It is best to take calcium around 2 hours before or after taking these and other drugs.

Avoid taking calcium citrate with aluminum-containing antacids. This combination has been seen to increase your body's absorption of aluminum. Aluminum has been associated with senility and Alzheimer's

Calcium is safe for pregnant women and they should take an adequate amount of calcium.

The best calcium to take is calcium citrate, gluconate, orotate or aspartate.

The gluconate type is similar to the calcium you get from milk and some vegetables. It is gentle calcium and is easily absorbed by children and adults with weak digestion.

The foods to eat for good calcium are:

Goat milk, egg yolk, fish, lemons, raw rhubarb, cheese, skimmed milk, bone broth, seeds, dulse, kelp, greens, nuts, cauliflower, celery, cottage cheese, gelatin preparations, bran,

Magnesium

Magnesium, a gentle laxative, helps to prevent constipation by relaxing your colon walls when you are under stress, have anxiety, or have too many worries. It normalizes tension on colon walls, allowing for a normal peristaltic action.

Because magnesium attracts water, you can bring in more water into your colon by taking magnesium supplements or by eating foods, which are high in magnesium. Water in your colon makes your stools softer and allows your colon to absorb water from your fecal matter if your body needs more water.

How do you know if you are short on magnesium? You will get cramps in your calves at night or so called "Charlie horses."

Or, you will feel sore after some mild exercise or activity.

Take 400 mg in the morning and 400 mg in the evening of Magnesium gluconate, or citrate.

11: What Fiber To Use For Constipation

What is Fiber?

Fiber is a carbohydrate that comes from cell walls and structure of plants, grains, legumes, fruits, and vegetables. Most processed or junk food has little fiber, since it is removed during processing.

Most people eat around 7-12 grams of fiber each day. You should be eating from 25 – 45 grams each day to prevent serious illnesses in your body.

A diet with 35 to 40 grams of fiber provides protection and prevention against diseases such as kidney stones, varicose veins, obesity, heart disease, appendicitis, colon disease, diabetes, appendicitis, diverticulosis, and many others.

When you eat fiber, it passes into your colon without getting digested in the small intestine. The good bacteria will use some of it as food, which makes them stronger and able to multiply.

Eating fiber reduces your fecal matter transit time from 3 days to 1 1/ 2 - 2days.

All processed food, such as white flour products, have little or no fiber. Fiber is removed when various natural flours or grains are processed to make junk food. During this processing, nutrients, vitamins, and minerals are also removed. Only plant foods and lightly processed grains have fiber of varying amounts

Foods that are "fortified" with vitamins and minerals are

unbalanced, since manufacturers cannot replace all the nutrients the food once had.

Fiber, bulk, or roughage, is one of the main nutrients you need to eat daily to relieve and prevent constipation and prevent many other diseases. Fiber is a nondigestible, complex carbohydrate. Most fiber is fermented in your colon and provides some energy for the body. Fiber has two forms – soluble and insoluble.

Eating Fiber

As you can see fiber is a critical nutrient for your colon and overall health. You need to eat equal amounts of insoluble and soluble fiber. Most people only eat around 10 grams or less of fiber each day.

You may experience gas when you start eating more fiber.

If you have any serious gastrointestinal illnesses, check with your doctor before adding more fiber to your diet.

One other major benefit of fiber is that, fiber stimulates pancreatic secretions - enzymes and bicarbonates - which help you to digest your food better and prevents undigested protein from reaching your colon.

When you are constipated, your fecal matter remains in contact with your colon walls longer. Undigested protein that is embedded in the fecal matter starts to decompose and putrefies. This undigested protein and putrid matter serves to feed bad bacteria and changes your colon environment into a toxic generator.

If you have not been eating a lot of fiber in the form of vegetable, fruits and grains, you need to add these foods to your eating habits little by little, so your body gets use to more fiber.

The more fiber you eat the more vitamins and minerals are lost and eliminated in your stools. What this means, is you need to compensate for this loss by eating more nutritious foods and or by using supplements.

Provide yourself with natural forms of fiber, such as vegetables, fruits, and legumes. Stay away from the supplemental forms of fiber such as, powders or pills. These pills may help in relieving constipation, but do little to provide you with nutrients found in good produce.

Supplemental fiber granules, powders, or pills can become addictive.

Limit your use of fiber that comes from grains. I know you have been told you need to eat a lot of bran, whole-wheat products, cereals, oats, oatmeal, buckwheat, unprocessed bran, rice bran, and so on.

In their recent book, 2001, Electrical Nutrition, Denie and Shelley Hiestand pointed out that our digestive system was not designed to process grains. When we eat food, our digestive system was designed to ferment food, to break it down, and make their nutrients available for our bodies. Then Hiestand's continues,

"Our digestive tract, like that of the grazing animals, is almost completely unable to ferment a seed-head (grain), whether it is whole or ground up as in flour...when we try to eat grain, the innate frequency of the seed-head can only go into storage—in other words, lay down cellulite...

This is why in agriculture to fatten up the hog or cattle, we feed them grain. Likewise, if you want to fatten up, eat grains... they take the most energy to digest, and we get little or nothing from it except large thighs, butts, and bellies.

REMEMBER THE OLD FARM SAYING GRAINS FOR GAIN,

PROTEIN FOR PRODUCTION. From an electrical nutrition perspective, modern grains could well be considered toxic."

Limit the use of grains to get your fiber. Make more use of vegetables, fruits, and legumes to get fiber.
However, when trying to clear constipation, fiber from bran can be used for a limited time.

Eating Bran

Eating bran is one of the quickest and best ways to increase your fiber. It will increase the weight and size of your stools more than the fiber contained in fruits or vegetables. Bran is the outer husk of the grain – wheat, corn, rice, and oat – which is indigestible.

It does not irritate the lining of the stomach, small intestine or your colon. It is not a laxative but promotes the movement fecal matter through your colon in a natural way. Unlike drugstore laxatives or other natural strong laxatives, bran does not quickly purge out all the contents in your colon.

Use one or two heaping tablespoon of bran in your morning cereal, in your baking, and in your smoothies.

When using bran, make sure you drink plenty of water, during the day to keep your stools soft.

Here are some other ways to use bran. You can add them to,

- baked breads, muffins and other baked goods
- breaded mixes
- hamburger meat
- juices
- pancake or waffle mix

- salads
- scramble eggs
- soups
- soups
- stuffing
- vegetarian burger mix
- yogurt

When you put bran in juices or anything that is all liquid, just eat it with a spoon.

How much bran should you take for good bowel regularity? Each person is different. You need to experiment. Start with two teaspoons each day and work towards 10 teaspoons a day or until you have bowel movements without effort or straining.

There are four basic bran products – wheat, corn, oat, and rice.

They all provide a solid source of fiber in varying amounts. Make sure the bran you use is 100% unprocessed bran.

Use bran for a few weeks to get your bowel movements back to normal. Eating bran should get your bowels moving in a few days or less.

Once your bowels are back to normal, back off from using a lot of bran and depend more on fiber from eating more fruits, vegetables, nuts, and seeds.

There are many new products, which use bran added to other nutrients or powders. Although these can be useful, use them for a limited time.

Wheat Bran

Many people use wheat bran to get more fiber in their diet. This was something that was encouraged in the past. But now you should limit or reduce the use of bran as a way to get more fiber in your diet.

Wheat bran is not the best bran to use but can be used in combination with oat, rice, or corn bran, which is better.

Wheat bran consists mainly of insoluble fiber. It consists of cellulose, hemi-cellulose, lignin, pectin, and pentosans. It absorbs plenty of water making the stools bulky and soft, which allows them to move through your colon easily. Bulky fiber stools help to scrub your colon walls to keep them clean of mucus and toxic build up.

Eating any bran requires drinking plenty of water throughout the day otherwise it can cause constipation.

When eating bran in any form, cereal, pancakes, or muffins, always drink extra water during the day. Bran absorbs water and becomes larger. Use water to help move it easily through your colon.

Young children should not eat wheat or rice bran. Eating bran requires drinking plenty of water throughout the day. Eating too much bran can cause the fecal matter to become too bulky and can cause constipation instead of relieving it.

Bran contains a high level of phytates, which interferes with absorption of calcium, zinc, iron and copper. For this reason, use a maximum of 1/3 of a cup of bran each day for yourself and for children use 1/6 of a cup. Excess use of wheat bran would require taking calcium, zinc, iron and copper supplements.

Bran is also high in B-vitamins and consists of around 21%

protein.

Children should not eat as much fiber as adults. Children should eat oat cereal, whole-grain cereals, fruits and vegetables.

Corn Bran

Corn bran has even more fiber than wheat bran by 40%. So, corn bran is excellent for prevent constipation. Both corn bran and wheat bran should be used in moderation and not used as the main ingredient in trying to prevent constipation. There is one concern with corn bran. Corn has been put on the list of GMO's. You may not want to feed your children corn that has been genetically modified. If you are pregnant, you may want to avoid.

Oat Bran

Oat bran has both soluble and insoluble fiber, which make its better to use than wheat bran. However, it does have less insoluble fiber than wheat and rice bran. It can be found with relatively little processing, which helps to maintain its high quality of protein, carbohydrates and vitamins.

Keep away of commercially made oat, wheat or other type of bran muffins since they contain a lot of fat, sugar and other additives that are unhealthy for you.

Rice Bran

For preventing constipation, rice bran is better than wheat bran.

In their book called High Speed Healing, 1991, the editor of Prevention Magazine Health Books, said that,

"You may see a dramatic improvement in your fight against

constipation by using rice bran- instead of wheat – to increase the size and frequency of your stools. One European study says that rice beats the living chaff out of wheat when it comes to fecal output and frequency of bowel movements."

Do not take your calcium supplement with bran Cereals, since fiber can interfere with calcium absorption.

Do not use cereal with bran in it. This bran has been processed and loses some of its fiber content. Use the bran sold as coarse granules. Add it to your morning cereals, smoothies, shakes, cottage cheese, yogurt, or other dishes.

12: How To Eat When You Have Constipation

Natural Body Cycles

Most of you are looking for ways to improve your health, lose weight, or get rid of an illness that you have. If you have acid reflux or heartburn, then you might be looking for a way to prevent it from coming back, after you have completed a colon cleanse.

Here's some information that will help you achieve these results. It is called "Using the Natural Body Cycles" for achieving maximum health.

By learning how to assist your "Natural Body Cycles", you will be in tune with what your body is doing to maintain your health.

Getting in tune with your Natural Body Cycles requires a change in the way you eat. Since all of us are addicted to the way we eat, it is, sometimes, difficult to change these habits. But if you are serious about what you want, this is the best information I have found that will give you great health.

By using this method to gain better health, you may experience some side effects, because you will be eliminating more body toxins and body wastes than normal. The side effects may be headaches, stomach upsets, body pain, or similar types of symptoms. These conditions will not last and will disappear as you get rid of more toxins. So if you experience these side effects, don't let them stop you from moving forward on this eating pattern.

Here are the 3 natural body cycles:

Cycle 1 time period: 4 am to noon

This cycle is the time where your body is eliminating toxins, acids, wastes, and derby by urine, bowel movements, sweating, and other secretions.

Cycle 2 time period: noon to 8 pm

This is the time when your body should be taking in solid and heavy food and digesting it.

Cycle 3 time period: 8 pm to 4 am.

This is the time your body is absorbing and using the food you have eaten during the noon to 8 pm period. It is the time your body is eliminating toxins from your body's organs and liquid and doing cell regeneration.

Only Cycle 1 will be discussed here since this is the time where you can make a big impact in eliminating constipation and getting your colon back to normal function.

Here's how to use cycle 1:

During the elimination cycle, 4 am to noon, eat and drink only fruits and their juices or drink vegetable juices. For breakfast eat a bowl of fruit or have a fruit smoothie made with apple juice and fruits in season. Before noontime, eat fruits as a snack. Forty-five minutes before noon eat your last fruit.
You can eat and drink all the fruits and juices you want up to noontime. Eat those fruits listed in the previous chapters and below.

Bananas, oranges, apricots, strawberries, melon, watermelons, apples, peaches, nectarines, and so on.

Eat all melons together and not with another fruit and wait ½ hour before eating other fruits. Melons require their specific enzymes to be digested in the stomach so other fruit eaten with melons will just sit in your stomach waiting to be digested.

By eating in this way you are assisting your body's elimination cycle. This helps your body to eliminate toxins and acids from your body and blood. It is these toxins and acids that make you sick, overweight, and cause constipation.

Eating solid food for breakfast – eggs potatoes, rice, meat, cereal, milk, and so on - interfere with your body's elimination cycle and eventually leads to sickness and excess weight. On occasion, you can eat cereal with fruit for variation.

It takes over three hours to digest heavy and solid food. The food you should be eating, in the morning, should digest quickly to help remove toxins, acids, and waste from your body.

Heavy food slows down the elimination of toxins from your body, and this causes more toxins to remain in the body, which get stored as fats and acids. Acids are the main cause of most illnesses, and so you want to have an alkaline body. Fruits and vegetables give you an alkaline body.
It takes ½ to 1 ½ hours to digest fruits and fruit juices. Because of this, they help to cleanse your body of waste and activate peristaltic action. Fruits are 70% water just like your body.

So if you are not already having fruit and fruit juices for breakfast and snacks, start slowing changing your habits, if you want to eliminate constipation, lose weight and feel better.

Herbal tea

The morning is also good for drinking herbal tea. As soon as you get up, make fresh ginger tea mixed with a green tea bag and a slight bit of honey. Drink one glass in the morning and one during the day or evening.

Now, one other thing, don't eat fruits and juices after lunch or dinner meals.

Last Meal For The Day

Eat your last meal by 6-7pm so that your food digests in your stomach by the time you go to bed. After three hours later, your food will have moved into your small intestine where it is ready for assimilation

When you go to bed 3 hours after your last meal, the next 6 hours, until 4am, your body will be absorbing the food you have eaten the previous day.

13: Resources You Need To Know About

Get one of my best kindle books *free* below:

http://www.natural-remedies-thatwork.com

Rudy Silva is a natural nutritional consultant educated in the United States in Nutrition and Physics. He is a graduate from San Jose State University in California. He is author of 45 other books on natural remedies. He has authored a newsletter in natural remedies for over 10 years.

Resource page

Here are some of the other kindle e-books about natural remedies that have been written by this author. You can see the entire list at:

http://tinyurl.com/b2f7wd3

Acne Remedies
- Best natural acne treatments: Acne facial
- Effective Acne Treatments That Work

Constipation Remedies
- The Best Constipation Remedies
- Best Constipated Women Natural Cures
- How To Relieve Constipation With Fruits

Essential Fatty Acids
- Taking The Mystery Out Of Essential Fatty acids
- Amazing Fish Oil Benefits Revealed
- Omega 3 and 6 Mystery Exposed

Nutrition Remedies

- Updated Version - Secret Diet And Nutrition
- Secret Healthy Fruit Practices Revealed
- Fast Healing Juice Nutrition Therapy: Nutrition Tips 3
- Fantastic Alkaline Fruit Benefits Revealed
- Calcium (Discover How To Use Calcium To Avoid Devastating Diseases)
- Magnesium Nutrition Revealed
- Best Nutrition Health Practices

Stomach Remedies

- Acid Reflux: Fast and Easy Cures For Acid Reflux
- Asthma Treatment Cures With Remedies
- How To Do Natural Colon Cleansing
- Gastrointestinal Digestion Secrets Revealed

Misc Remedies

- Natural Hair Loss Treatment: Women And Men
- Effective Natural Hemorrhoids Treatment
- Iron Deficiency Anemia
- What Is A Hiatus Hernia
- Best Varicose Vein Treatments?
- How To Fix Your Thyroid Problems: Discover Hidden Ideas That Fix Your Thyroid
- Nail Fungus & Health Treatment: Fix Your Fingernail's Health And Look Beautiful
- Gout Diet: New Ideas For Gout Treatments and Gout remedies for Eliminating Uric Acid and giving Gout Relief
- Diarrhea: How To Stop Diarrhea Chronic Or Severe

Minerals

- The Magic of Sodium, Calcium and Magnesium
- Create an Alkaline Body with Potassium and Sodium: Eliminate a Potassium Deficiency

- Calcium and Phosphorus Foods: Deficiency or Excesses in These Minerals Cause Bone and Brain Power Loss

Men's Health
- Best Impotence Health Diet

Weight loss
- Ten (10) Day Quick Success Weight Loss Program: A new approach to losing weight by changing your eating habits for life
- Discover Secret Anti-Aging Juice & Tonic Recipes: Unique Juices And Tonics That Create Beauty And Youth

To see all of the kindle books written by this author, go to this the Authors Profile Page or this URL:

http://tinyurl.com/b2f7wd3

If you need support or want to promote any of his e-books, please contact him at rss41@yahoo.com and expect a reply within 24 hours. He looks forward to hearing from you and is happy to help you understand his material on natural and nutritional health.

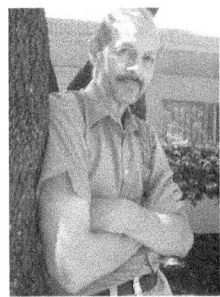

Give A Review

And, don't for get to give a review for this e-book at Amazon so that others can gain the benefits of what is in this e-book. To you, for losing weight, creating better health and more happiness in your life,

Rudy S Silva